Embrace Bravery

Embracing Your Infertility Story
with Bravery and Strength

Shannon Ketchum

Table of Contents

Endorsements by Beth Forbus, Jeanne Mayo,
Geri Alicea & Kayla Dawson

Dedication

To Father God – to the giver of life, the One who has never given up on me, who has amazing plans for my life and truly does immeasurably more than I can imagine – I devote this book to your glory. Thank you for loving me and for giving the best for me.

To my amazing husband – your patience through this journey has never gone unnoticed. Your support means more than you will ever know. And your love makes me one of the luckiest women in the world. I love, cherish and adore you, babe.

Mom, Dad, Renee & Desiree – I love you immensely. We've had so many adventures together as a family, and I wouldn't trade any of it. Thank you for always seeking to understand what I've been through in the midst of dealing with delayed fertility and supporting me. You have given me the strength to continue moving forward. Mom & Dad, thanks for always leading me to Christ and setting me up for success in life.

To Sugar Hill Baptist Support Group – Anna, Dana, Ashley, Jen, Mandy, Marcey – my sisters, you gave me a place to really process some of the hardest moments in my fertility journey. You helped me to realize that I wasn't alone in this journey and helped support God's calling on my life to encourage women in their own fertility journeys. You will never know the impact you truly have had on my life.

Dennis & Colleen Rouse, thanks for your vision for Victory Church and your staff. Thanks for believing in me as part of your team and giving me a place to call home for so many years. The training I've received at Victory in ministry, in small groups and in marketing, all have prepared me for the season of life I'm in now. I will always be grateful to you for that. **Pam Parish**, thank you for giving me my start at Victory, thanks for believing in me and thank you for your support. I loved being your assistant and I'm blessed to know you! The work you're doing with Connections Homes is so amazing! **Michael Buckingham**, Thanks for always believing in me and supporting me and encouraging me to go higher in ministry. Your support has meant the world to me. **Gladys & Pete Torres**, thank you for your friendship and for your mentorship over the years. You have impacted not only my life, my work but also my marriage in ways you will never truly know. And a special thanks for your prayers and support in our transition to Florida. **Raegan Carlson**, I'm beyond thankful for your friendship. You're an amazing listener and oh so supportive! I love how happy you always are for me as things have transpired within my personal life and my ministry. I love you, Rae! **Nathan Davis + Ty Buckingham**, I'm beyond thankful to both of you for everything you've done to support me and the *Embrace Bravery* ministry. Thanks for believing in me and my vision. It means more than you know!

To some of the best friends a girl could ask for – Kelly Baker, it's now been 13 years that we've been friends since we first shared that one plate of chicken tenders together at Chili's – who knew then that we would have created a lifelong friendship? You are a true bestie! You've been there for all my biggest moments in life – whether they've been good or bad! I'm so blessed to call you my bestie! You're an amazing person and an amazing friend! And I just know God has some amazing things planned for your life! Thanks for always supporting me! I love you, Kel Kel! **Jeannelle Higgins**, who knew when I first met you – and I didn't like you, ha! – that we would become so close? Only God! He had some amazing plans up His sleeves for us! You've been a true sister friend! And I'm so blessed by your friendship. I just love how no matter what's going on in your world, you always find the strength to be happy for me. Your support... there are no words to describe what it means. I love you, sis! **Leah Hoverman**, a chance encounter at a small group meeting after your hubby introduced us... God knew what He was up to! This sweet friendship we've developed over the last two years has been awesome. And to make it even sweeter, our hubby's are great friends, too! I love that we have such a sweet couple friendship! The fact that God gave me another infertility sister to become besties with just shows how amazing our God is! So grateful for your friendship, support, and assistance with *Embrace Bravery*. I can't wait to see what God does with *Rebekah's Rose*! Love you, my friend!

Ladies of Embrace Bravery – I dedicate this book to all of you in *Embrace Bravery* now and those who will be in the future – you are why I'm doing ministry and writing this book! Thanks for your bravery – to step forward and share with others your stories of loss and pain – there's no one stronger! I'm standing with you and believing with you – immeasurably more than you can imagine will be yours!

Endorsements

A few times in a lifetime, we encounter a book that powerfully mirrors the author's own deepest challenges and raw vulnerability. If you just picked up Shannon Ketchum's priceless book, **Embrace Bravery**, you have found this rare kind of book. Shannon courageously unwraps her story of infertility and gives a genuine lifeline to couples struggling with this challenge. It is a brilliant, transparent, inspiring, and yet highly practical book on one of the most challenging problems a woman will ever face. And sadly enough, even in the church world, she often feels she must face this "looming cloud" all alone. I simply cannot recommend **Embrace Bravery** highly enough.

— DR. JEANNE MAYO, *Author and public speaker, Founder & President of The Cadre, Founder & President of Youth Leader's Coach, Director of Youth & Young Adult Ministries at Victory Church in Norcross GA & Executive Director of Atlanta Leadership College*

Embrace Bravery walks you through the struggles of infertility and helps bring you to a place of hopeful expectation. As I read, I could feel tiny seeds of hope being planted in the soil of my heart. I felt encouraged and so much lighter after working through this book. Shannon spoke to the hard feelings I am struggling with and gave me permission to work through those feelings with God. She really understood my heart and her encouraging, God-given words helped me to be kinder to myself.

— KAYLA DAWSON, *Embrace Bravery Launch Team Member*

Embrace Bravery is a must-read for any woman dealing with infertility. Read this book and gain practical tips on how to embrace your journey with bravery and courage.

— GERI ALICEA, *Founder of Womb Prep & Embrace Bravery Launch Team Member*

Foreword

by Beth Forbus,
Founder of Sarah's Laughter

What an honor to speak on behalf of Shannon Ketchum and **Embrace Bravery.**

Embrace Bravery is more than just a book. It is a lifeline for those walking the life-changing journey of infertility. Author Shannon Ketchum leads the reader on an interactive journey through the ups and downs of infertility, placing weapons in your hand to enable you to fight the battles of discouragement, fear, and worry.

Intertwined within Shannon's personal story of delayed fertility are abundant Scriptures, pointing you toward the truth of God's Word rather than the lies infertility tries to deposit into you. This book conveys what your heart has felt but couldn't find the words to say. Power statements help you not only remember what you've read but apply it to your journey as well. Support groups will find this work a valuable asset to their meetings with discussion guides and topics.

This narrative is a must-have for every couple on the journey through unwanted childlessness.

Introduction
My Story & Where This Begins

Maybe you've picked up this book and the title intrigues you, but you have no idea who this chick, Shannon Ketchum is. Allow me to tell you why you should continue to read on and how I can relate to pieces of your own infertility story.

I've been married to my amazing husband, Carl, since 2003 and together we share a life in Tallahassee, FL with our fur babies — pit bull mixes, Jackson & Sydney and Pomeranian, Reno. All of these babies are the light of my life! And my fur babies definitely keep me entertained.

My husband and I knew right away that there was something wrong in our sex and fertility journey. You see, I was having excruciating pain during sex ... to the point of screaming and crying in pain. We gave it some time, as I wasn't ready to really let someone into this private area of our life. So after about a year, I started seeking the help of our GYN. She told me I could have an internal ultrasound to find out if there was anything to be concerned about. I should mention that even my annual women's exams were so painful that I would scream and cry. So, an internal ultrasound was kind of scary to me.

After I had that done, the next step was to have a laparoscopy to see if they could find anything like endometriosis. For those that don't know, this is a surgery that comes with a painful recovery. I decided to hold off for about a year because surgery was very scary to me.

Meanwhile, the reality of not being able to get pregnant was really starting to sink in. At this point, I started getting pretty sad that it hadn't happened for us and wondering what's wrong with me. Am I so defective that I can't have a child? I went through moments of anger, sadness, and very low self-esteem. I couldn't believe this was my reality, as all I ever wanted growing up was to be a mom, and it wasn't happening the way it was supposed to. My body's failing me. I was created to have babies, and it's not happening. Does any of this sound like some of what you've been saying?

After a year had passed, I went through the very painful laparoscopy. I come out of it to find I've been diagnosed with endometriosis and they scraped what they found off of my uterus. Oh, and in addition, I also have a condition called pelvic engorgement syndrome which basically means there are blood vessels growing around my pelvis causing all of the pain during cycles and sex. My doctor then explains that there is no cure for this, but there is a doctor doing some experimental procedures that might work. I was devastated. No cure. I thought I was finally going to have answers.

After I took a few months to process through my grief, I decided to move forward with the experimental procedure. After I woke up from my surgery, they told me "You don't have this condition. I don't know what your doctor saw, but you don't have it." I was even more devastated. I would even say I was broken. I didn't want this condition, but at least I had answers, and I thought this would at least give me a temporary cure. But no, again another fork in the road on this journey. At this point, I'm about 5-6 years into my fertility journey.

Shortly after that, I was diagnosed with polycystic ovarian syndrome (PCOS), another condition that made getting pregnant a challenge. Oh, and I forgot to mention that I was also diagnosed with hypothyroidism, which also impacted my fertility.

After all of this, feeling broken and damaged, I found out my sister was pregnant with her second child. This news devastated me. It contributed to putting me in a dark place of depression and despair. I didn't really want to talk to anyone. I didn't want to go to church. I didn't want to pray. I didn't want to hear any encouraging words. I just wanted to grieve and mourn. I was mad, I was angry, I was frustrated. How could God who promised me years before that I would have children not be delivering? How could He be giving everyone else children? How come I had to watch everyone else? Did You mean it when You promised me? I doubted what He had told me. I never doubted that He was God or that He was good. I just doubted that He was good to *me*.

After about a year of being like this, I had had enough. I couldn't live like this anymore. In fact, this isn't living.

I started talking to a counselor at my church, and this woman really helped launch me into the beginning stages of processing through my pain. Because of that, I was able to start attending a local infertility support group at my mother's church. This place finally gave me a place to deal with my pain and gave me sisters who understood what I was going through. This is where my healing began.

While participating in the infertility group, I also started seeing a new doctor. With this new doctor, I had to share my fertility story all over again. She attempted an exam and couldn't finish because the pain was so bad that I was crying and screaming. So, she did two things: 1. She believed I had a muscle spasm condition, and ordered physical therapy. 2. She wanted to confirm the PCOS diagnosis and start treating it.

When she said physical therapy, I swear I looked at her like she had bananas coming out of her ears. Therapy for that?!?!? Yes, therapy for that. Through physical therapy, I finally had a confirmed diagnosis for my pain 'pelvic dysfunction'. My pelvis didn't lay in the right position, therefore causing all my pain. So we've been on a journey to strengthen and relax my pelvis. All of this came at about 12 years into my marriage and fertility journey. Yes, it took 12 years to have a diagnosis. Finally, I knew I wasn't crazy. I knew I hadn't invented this pain in my head. There's not something wrong with me as a person. There's something wrong physically, and now I finally had answers.

I shared all of this with my support group and they were just as shocked as I was. But more importantly, one of the ladies said, "You are so brave." Brave? What? Me?!? I didn't really believe it.

SHANNON KETCHUM

Several months later, my husband sent me on an infertility retreat with 30 other women. Just getting there was all God. But while there, God spoke to me so clearly. After sharing my story, one of the women said, "You are so brave". I'm thinking, really? This is the second person to say this to me. Maybe there's something to this. Then, I found this cup on a table of mugs to choose from and mine said, "Be you bravely." I was really beginning to believe there was something to this "brave" thing.

As the retreat continued the Lord began to tell me, "You are brave. You are not broken. My promises are still good for you. I have not forgotten you. You can believe in me. You can have hope. You can trust me, I will not disappoint you." I was undone by Him. This is the moment when the Lord truly healed my heart of the pain and grief of infertility. It was the moment I stopped doubting and truly started to believe His plans for my life and my family's life.

From this point, it's where my women's ministry, *Embrace Bravery* was born. A ministry for women with infertility was launched in April of 2017. This ministry is all about offering support to other women dealing with infertility and loss, a place where we can learn to bravely embrace our infertility journey and begin to trust God in the midst of our waits for our family. I've been afforded the opportunity to dig into women's lives, support them and encourage them via support groups, social media, my blog, now this book and speaking engagements. It's truly not something I expected to be doing, but it's one of the best things I've ever been able to do.

It's from this place that this book was birthed. I want to help you bravely embrace your journey.

In each chapter, I have created a space for you to create a power statement — an affirmation you're choosing to speak over yourself of what you've learned from the chapter. I want to equip you with resources for these power statements. So, in this book you will find a few ways to utilize your power statements:

1. Write it in the power statement section in each chapter.
2. With your phone, take a picture of the QR code in Appendix B at the back of this book to download a power statement graphic that you can use as a template on your phone to create a graphic yourself with your power statement.

xvi

This book was specifically designed with support groups in mind. If you're leading a support group through this material, check out the Appendix A at the back of the book for more details on how to best use this book.

Won't you come along with me — maybe even grab a few girlfriends to do this along with you? Stay for a while, spend time in the Word, lift your prayers and your grief to the Lord. Learn what it looks like to be brave in the face of infertility.

> *Yet the Lord longs to be gracious to you; therefore he will rise up to show you compassion. For the Lord is a God of justice. Blessed are all who wait for him!* — Isaiah 30:18 NIV

> *Now to him who is able to do immeasurably more than all we ask or imagine, according to his power that is at work within us...* — Ephesians 3:20 NIV

Praying with you,
Shannon

1

Infertility vs. Fertility

Infertility. Have you been labeled with that word? I know I have. And it begins to define us. Unable to conceive. Unable to produce. Broken. Not worthy of motherhood. Maybe these are some of the words you've used to describe yourself or started to believe because of this label someone put on you.

Both broken and not worthy of motherhood are two pieces of that label that I identified with most. You know what happened? I was believing those things and not even realizing it. It took God reaching in and showing me the truth for me to realize it.

You're not broken.

First, He showed me that I'm not broken. I may have broken pieces, but that doesn't mean I'm broken. The broken pieces in my life (infertility being one of them) are what He's using to add onto my story and cause me to move forward. He will use those pieces for His glory. He will use them for the benefit of my story helping others. Doesn't that just give a sweet purpose to the pain?

Well, I'll tell you one thing, when God first told me I was going to have a testimony from my story, I didn't want it. In fact, I told Him so. I told Him, "I don't want your stupid testimony, I just want a baby." It might sound harsh, but that's how I was feeling. Is that how you're feeling too? Don't worry, that's totally okay if that's how you feel. Our feelings are important for us to process through and deal with.

But you know what, as God began to peel back different layers of my story, I began to see my story as beautiful and something I wanted to use to help others. I think He'll do the same for you.

You are worthy of being a mom.

Second, He showed me that I felt like He was saying I wasn't worthy of motherhood. Wait.... what?!?!? Yes, He really did tell me that and it completely threw me off. You know why it threw me off? Because I didn't even know I felt that way. As I dug into further conversation with God, He showed me that because I didn't have children yet, I felt like He was saying I wasn't worthy to be a mom. Whoa! Right?!!??

The truth of the matter is this: that couldn't be further from the truth. He designed us all to be mothers, no matter what things are currently standing in our way. Family is part of the DNA of who God is. I mean just look at Adam and Eve. He created family starting with them.

Your words

Can I tell you something? It's time that we start speaking life over ourselves and our wombs instead of death. Proverbs 18 in the Message version says:

> *"Words kill, words give life; they're either poison or fruit—you choose."*

I don't know about you, but I want fruit, not poison. I don't want to poison my mind or my body with words. I want to empower my mind and body with my words. Let's vow to do that today.

Dr. Caroline Leaf, a cognitive neuroscientist, says the following about toxic thoughts:

> *The average person has over 30,000 thoughts a day. Through an uncontrolled thought life, we create the conditions for illness; we make ourselves sick! Research shows that fear, all on its own, triggers more than 1,400 known*

physical and chemical responses and activates more than 30 different hor-
mones. There are INTELLECTUAL and MEDICAL reasons to FORGIVE!
Toxic waste generated by toxic thoughts causes the following illnesses: diabetes,
cancer, asthma, skin problems, and allergies to name just a few. Consciously
control your thought life and start to detox your brain!

Medical research increasingly points to the fact that thinking and consciously
controlling your thought life is one of the best ways, if not the best way of detox-
ing your brain. It allows you to get rid of those toxic thoughts and emotions that
can consume and control your mind.[1]

If this is how our thoughts affect us, imagine how the actual words that form
from our thoughts affect us. Because when we speak those words, we're giving
even more power to them.

So let's start with the first positive words about our journey:

I am fertile.

How does that feel when you say that? Does it feel weird? Does it feel right?
It was weird at first for me because I thought I was saying something false.
But you know what, I'm not saying something that's not right. I'm actually
claiming and speaking these words over myself. I am fertile. I will produce.
Because when we say that do you know who we're giving power to? We're no
longer giving power to the enemy. We're giving power to God. He has more
power than we realize. But now, when I say it it feels right, it's because I'm
saying God can and will do it.

Your Identity

What does God say about us? Who are we really? Because we are not infertility.
That may be a part of our story, but it doesn't define us.

Here's what defines us:

I am a child of God.
But to all who have received him—those who believe in his name—he has given
the right to become God's children ... (John 1:12 NET)[2]

I have been accepted by Christ.
Receive one another, then, just as Christ also received you, to God's glory.
(Romans 15:7 NET)[2]

My body is a temple of the Holy Spirit who dwells in me.
Do you not know that you are God's temple and that God's Spirit lives in you?
(1 Corinthians 6:19 NET)[2]

I am a new creature in Christ.
So then, if anyone is in Christ, he is a new creation; what is old has passed away—look, what is new has come! (2 Corinthians 5:17 NET)[2]

I have been blessed with every spiritual blessing in the heavenly places.
Blessed is the God and Father of our Lord Jesus Christ, who has blessed us with every spiritual blessing in the heavenly realms in Christ. (Ephesians 1:3 NET)[2]

I am chosen, holy, and blameless before God.
For he chose us in Christ before the foundation of the world that we may be holy and unblemished in his sight in love. (Ephesians 1:4 NET)[2]

I have boldness and confident access to God through faith in Christ.
… In whom we have boldness and confident access to God because of Christ's faithfulness. (Ephesians 3:12 NET)[2]

The peace of God guards my heart and mind.
And the peace of God that surpasses all understanding will guard your hearts and minds in Christ Jesus. (Philippians 4:7 NET)[2]

I have been chosen of God, and I am holy and beloved.
Therefore, as the elect of God, holy and dearly loved, clothe yourselves with a heart of mercy, kindness, humility, gentleness, and patience …
(Colossians 3:12 NET)[2]

God loves me and has chosen me.

We know, brothers and sisters loved by God, that he has chosen you ... (1 Thessalonians 1:4 NET)[2]

I am God's incredible work of art.

For we are God's handiwork, created in Christ Jesus to do good works, which God prepared in advance for us to do. (Ephesians 2:10 NIV)[3]

I am greatly loved.

But God demonstrates his own love for us in this: While we were still sinners, Christ died for us. (Romans 5:8 NIV)[3]

For I am convinced that neither death nor life, neither angels nor demons, neither the present nor the future, nor any powers, neither height nor depth, nor anything else in all creation, will be able to separate us from the love of God that is in Christ Jesus our Lord. (Romans 8:38-39 NIV)

I am worth more than jewels.

A wife of noble character who can find? She is worth far more than rubies. (Proverbs 31:10 NIV)

I am fearfully and wonderfully made.

For you created my inmost being; you knit me together in my mother's womb. I praise you because I am fearfully and wonderfully made; your works are wonderful, I know that full well. My frame was not hidden from you when I was made in the secret place when I was woven together in the depths of the earth. Your eyes saw my unformed body; all the days ordained for me were written in your book before one of them came to be. How precious to me are your thoughts, God! How vast is the sum of them! Were I to count them, they would outnumber the grains of sand—when I awake, I am still with you. (Psalm 139:13-18 NIV)

Do you see what God says about you? Do you see your value and worth? I especially want to stay on *"I am fearfully and wonderfully made"*. This one specifically is so powerful to us, as women. Not just because of fertility challenges. As women, we have such a hard time with our esteem, beauty, and worth. On top of that, we often feel like we are a mistake because of infertility. But do you see what God says here? I am wonderfully made! Not a mistake, not broken, not ugly. I am wonderfully made by the Creator of the universe. He saw it as part of His perfect plan and design to create me.

> "I would rather be what God chose to make me than the most glorious creature that I could think of; for to have been thought about, born in God's thought, and then made by God, is the dearest, grandest and most precious thing in all thinking." — **George MacDonald**

Power Statement

This is a brief statement (similar to an affirmation) that you're setting for yourself of what you will choose to believe about your fertility.

I choose

_____

_____

Questions for discussion:

1. Have you ever felt that you are broken? Why or why not?
2. Have you ever felt unworthy for motherhood? Why or why not?
3. What can you do to begin changing the words you speak in order to speak fruit instead of poison?
4. Read Galatians 4:27. Do you see the benefits we will have after being barren for our journey? Does that get you excited that we have something that no one else has?

2

Bravery

Brave. How does that word make you feel? Do you hate it? Do you like it? You know how I felt about that word? I hated it with everything in me. Do you know why? My introverted personality made me feel weak, anxious, fearful, and just plain terrified. Then, you add on top of that my fertility journey and that just magnifies feeling the opposite of bravery.

The definition of brave according to dictionary.com is "possessing or exhibiting courage or courageous endurance". So, what is courage then? Courage is defined as "the quality of mind or spirit that enables a person to face difficulty, danger, pain, etc. without fear." (www.dictionary.com) In other words, being brave means you have the ability to face pain or difficulty without fear.

I asked some friends and family what "brave" meant to them and here are some of their thoughts:

- Facing your fears boldly no matter how scared you are.
- Stepping out of what makes you comfortable even when you don't feel like it.

- Choosing to look confidently toward the future even though I don't know what it holds. And I choose to give my all, even though I may fail.
- Doing what you hear God telling you to do even if it is against the grain, is at cost or doesn't make sense.
- Doing things or going through obstacles that you might not like but you have to. It's going places that no one else is daring to go. Sometimes it means being quiet and letting God tell you what you really need to do and to listen and obey.

For me, being brave means that I trust fully in Him to lead me through everything, even the very scary and uncertain things.

Take Courage

> *Immediately Jesus made the disciples get into the boat and go on ahead of him to the other side, while he dismissed the crowd. After he had dismissed them, he went up on a mountainside by himself to pray. Later that night, he was there alone, and the boat was already a considerable distance from land, buffeted by the waves because the wind was against it. Shortly before dawn, Jesus went out to them, walking on the lake. When the disciples saw him walking on the lake, they were terrified. "It's a ghost," they said and cried out in fear. But Jesus immediately said to them: "Take courage! It is I. Don't be afraid." "Lord, if it's you," Peter replied, "Tell me to come to you on the water." "Come," he said. Then Peter got down out of the boat, walked on the water and came toward Jesus. But when he saw the wind, he was afraid and, beginning to sink, cried out, "Lord, save me!" Immediately Jesus reached out his hand and caught him. "You of little faith," he said, "why did you doubt?" And when they climbed into the boat, the wind died down. Then those who were in the boat worshiped him, saying, "Truly you are the Son of God."*
> *– Matthew 14:22-33 NIV*

Did you see that Jesus told them to "take courage"? Why would he say that to the disciples? Do you know what he was telling them? Take the position of being able to face the difficulty without fear. So He wanted them to let go of fear and face this situation head-on.

Then, a few moments later, Peter wanted to go out on the water with Jesus and walk on the water. And he did it! But what happened pretty quickly after he walked out on the water? He lost his faith and started to doubt and began to sink. Now if this isn't a true depiction of what happens with us, I don't know what is. We start out believing, we start with the courage, and then a moment later we start to doubt.

What can we learn from this passage?

1. The disciples had fear.

So even the disciples had fear. So if the cream-of-the-crop men that Jesus chose to walk with him were afraid, don't you think it's natural that we would be too? Fear is a pretty common thing. It's not something that's privy only to certain people. It's an all-encompassing thing for all of us.

Now we know that the disciples dealt with fear and that we all deal with it. Maybe we should understand it a little bit more. Merriam-Webster's dictionary describes fear as "an unpleasant often strong emotion caused by anticipation or awareness of danger, anxious concern or reason for alarm." So your fear is likely caused by anxiousness or anticipation of danger.

What is anxiousness or anxiety? Being anxious means being characterized by extreme uneasiness of mind. Maybe you are not at ease about something, but what does the Bible say about anxiety?

> *Cast all your anxiety on him because he cares for you.* — 1 Peter 5:7 NIV

> *Do not be anxious about anything, but in every situation, by prayer and petition, with thanksgiving, present your requests to God. And the peace of God, which transcends all understanding, will guard your hearts and your minds in Christ Jesus.* — Philippians 4:6-7 NIV

According to God's Word, we are called to give Him all of our cares, concerns, and anxiety. When we do so, He will give us peace. I have experienced this myself and it is so real. The peace He's talking about in Philippians is a supernatural peace that no one can explain. It's in moments that make no logical sense that we experience a peace that no one can explain. The only reason could be 'because God'.

2. Peter stepped out in the midst of fear.

Peter operated in this same line of thinking that I was talking about earlier, to do it afraid. He didn't really understand what Jesus was doing, but He knew He wanted to be where He was. I think many times, we for a moment decide to put our fear to the side and move forward.

How does it feel when we do that? Before the doubt creeps in, I think we might feel great, even accomplished. We should be because we didn't allow fear to get the best of us.

This is a place we need to live in. We need to push fear to the wayside and move forward despite our fear. Because what could potentially be waiting on the other side? Bigger and newer things that we may not have experienced otherwise. Even better, like Peter, Jesus could be waiting on the other end of that fear.

3. Peter doubted for a moment and gave into his fear again.

Peter doubted. And maybe like me, you initially criticized him. "How could you be doubting when you're looking at the face of Jesus? He's walking on the water, you're walking on the water. All is well." I know it's easy to criticize him during this moment. But really when you think about it, his response was completely normal. We all have a moment of weakness and forget what's in front of us. We all doubt. And you know what? It's okay. You know why? Because we have a Father who loves us, extends grace to us, and picks us up again. He might start out with asking why you doubted, but in the end, He'll pick you up because that's who He is.

—

All in all, we can learn that they feared, so we will fear. Peter let go of his fear and stepped out just like we can, and Peter doubted, just like we do. So now, we can take this and apply it to what I said bravery really is, fully trusting Him to lead me through everything... even the scary and uncertain things.

So what does that mean in the light of fertility challenges?

- When month after month, I don't get pregnant
- When I lose the baby
- When there's no explanation for my fertility challenges
- When there is an explanation that seems hopeless
- When the physical pain is unbearable
- When it's doctor's visit after doctor's visit
- When the money doesn't reach far enough for the medical bills or adoption preparation fees
- When IUI or IVF fails
- When adoption fails
- When I've lost all belief to hope

Those things seem unbearable like I just can't continue on. But you know what, God says His love never fails, He'll never leave us nor forsake us, that He has good plans for us, and that nothing is impossible with Him. So this tells me that I can choose to be brave in the face of fertility challenges; that I can trust Him, pray for His guidance, and move forward where He leads because He is a big God and He's bigger than my health problems or anything the doctors have to say. After all, He spoke and the universe came into existence, so that means He can speak my story into existence too. I just need to bravely believe in my big God.

Power Statement

This is a brief statement (similar to an affirmation) that you're setting for yourself of what you will choose to believe about yourself in regards to bravery.

I choose

_____

_____

Questions for discussion:

1. What does bravery look like to you?
2. Do you feel brave? Why or why not?
3. Read 2 Samuel 10:12 and 1 Chronicles 19:13. What do you notice? Why do you think this scripture is in the Bible twice? What does the Lord say He will do in these scriptures?
4. What are you afraid of? Does your fear debilitate you?

Brave

Moriah Peters, Brave, 2014, Reunion Records ©

No one ever told me this would be easy
But I never knew that it could be this hard
Oh the worry the worry the worry
Is weighing on me
Could you help me break down
All these question marks
And make me
I'll fight like a soldier
(Brave) rise like a warrior
(Brave) won't stop till the final day
(Brave) I want to be stronger
(Brave) gonna be bolder
(Brave) look up and I see the way
You make me brave
I know I know I'm no superwoman
But impossible is possible with you
So no, no, no more running, no more hiding
Strike the fire so I'll be fearless too
And make me
I'll fight like a soldier
(Brave) rise like a warrior
(Brave) won't stop till the final day
(Brave) I want to be stronger
(Brave) gonna be bolder
(Brave) look up and I see the way
You make me brave
None go with me
Still I'll follow
Through the joy

SHANNON KETCHUM

And through the sorrow
Cross before me
World behind me
There's no turning back

Songwriters: Brownleewe Matt / Moriah Peters / Joel Smallbone

3

Waiting

Waiting. Does anyone really like it? Does anyone really have the patience of waiting mastered? Is waiting hard for you? Do you hate it as much as I do?

Inevitably, waiting is something we will deal with in life. Waiting in traffic. Waiting in line at the grocery store. Waiting for the person you're going to marry to reveal themselves. Waiting for the dream job. Waiting for a baby. There are many seasons of waiting. Some are big and some are small. But why do we have to wait all the time? Is there a good reason for it? Is it just to torture us?

1. God acts on our behalf when we wait.

> *For since the beginning of the world men have not heard nor perceived by the ear, nor has the eye seen any God besides You, who acts for the one who waits for Him.* — Isaiah 64:4 NKJV

Isaiah 64:4 shows us that when we wait on God, He will act on our behalf. So even though it may seem like absolutely nothing happens while we wait,

God is doing things on our behalf while we wait. Sometimes it's things we can see and sometimes it's things we can't. But the only way it'll ever be revealed is if we allow Him to act on our behalf while we wait on Him to do His part.

2. God gives us new strength when we wait on Him.

But those who wait on the Lord shall renew their strength; they shall mount up with wings like eagles, They shall run and not be weary, they shall walk and not faint. — Isaiah 40:31 NKJV

Wait on the Lord; be of good courage, and He shall strengthen your heart; wait, I say, on the Lord! — Psalm 27:14 NKJV

Often times when we're waiting we lose our strength, we become tired. We exhaust ourselves. We become undone by our wait. How much longer can we do this and just wait and wait and wait??? But here God is telling us that you don't have to feel or live that way. He tells us if we wait on Him instead of looking at our circumstances He will renew us. He will give us new strength, and we won't feel run down or tired by the things around us. We will be able to rise to new heights that we've never been able to do before.

3. God helps us and protects us during our wait.

I will wait for You, O You his Strength; For God is my defense. — Psalm 59:9 NKJV

Our soul waits for the Lord; He is our help and our shield. — Psalm 33:20 NKJV

I waited patiently for the Lord, And He inclined to me, and heard my cry. — Psalm 40:1 NKJV

Do you often feel like you're alone in this? There's no one there to help you or protect you when harm comes your way? Well, we are so fortunate because God can be and is that help and protection for us! When we are hurting, when we are struggling, when we feel alone, He's there to help us through it and comfort us. When we feel danger coming our way, He will shield us from it. He's the God of angel armies! He's our warrior and we can feel safe in His arms!

4. We can rely on Him and wait expectantly.

> *My soul, wait silently for God alone, for my expectation is from Him.*
> —Psalm 62:5 NKJV

We can lift our requests to the God who put the stars in the sky, the God who spoke and breathed life into us, the God who chose us for a specific purpose, and the God who sacrificed His only Son to save us. That God is our God we can rely on and believe when we leave something at His feet, He hears us. It may not be answered or happen right at that moment, but we can know that we can wait expectantly for Him to do His work.

The Importance of Waiting on God

> *But Abram said, "Sovereign Lord, what can you give me since I remain child-less and the one who will inherit my estate is Eliezer of Damascus?" And Abram said, "You have given me no children; so a servant in my household will be my heir." Then the word of the Lord came to him: "This man will not be your heir, but a son who is your own flesh and blood will be your heir." He took him out-side and said, "Look up at the sky and count the stars—if indeed you can count them." Then he said to him, "So shall your offspring be." Abram believed the Lord, and he credited it to him as righteousness ... Now Sarai, Abram's wife, had borne him no children. But she had an Egyptian slave named Hagar; so she said to Abram, "The Lord has kept me from having children. Go, sleep with my slave; perhaps I can build a family through her." Abram agreed to what Sarai said. So after Abram had been living in Canaan ten years, Sarai his wife took her Egyptian slave Hagar and gave her to her husband to be his wife. He slept*

*with Hagar, and she conceived. When she knew she was pregnant, she began
to despise her mistress. Then Sarai said to Abram, "You are responsible for the
wrong I am suffering. I put my slave in your arms, and now that she knows
she is pregnant, she despises me. May the Lord judge between you and me." ...
Abraham looked up and saw three men standing nearby. When he saw them,
he hurried from the entrance of his tent to meet them and bowed low to the
ground ... "Where is your wife Sarah?" they asked him. "There, in the tent,"
he said. Then one of them said, "I will surely return to you about this time next
year, and Sarah your wife will have a son." Now Sarah was listening at the
entrance to the tent, which was behind him. Abraham and Sarah were already
very old, and Sarah was past the age of childbearing. So Sarah laughed to
herself as she thought, "After I am worn out and my lord is old, will I now have
this pleasure?" Then the Lord said to Abraham, "Why did Sarah laugh and
say, 'Will I really have a child, now that I am old?' Is anything too hard for the
Lord? I will return to you at the appointed time next year, and Sarah will have
a son." ... Now the Lord was gracious to Sarah as he had said, and the Lord
did for Sarah what he had promised. Sarah became pregnant and bore a son
to Abraham in his old age, at the very time God had promised him. Abraham
gave the name Isaac to the son Sarah bore him. When his son Isaac was eight
days old, Abraham circumcised him, as God commanded him. Abraham was a
hundred years old when his son Isaac —was born to him. Sarah said, "God has
brought me laughter, and everyone who hears about this will laugh with me."
And she added, "Who would have said to Abraham that Sarah would nurse
children? Yet I have borne him a son in his old age."*
— Genesis 15:2-6, 16:1-5, 18:2, 9-14, 21: 1-7 NIV

So here we see that God made a promise to Abraham and Sarah. They would
have a child and many descendants! How exciting to hear is that? To hear
from the God of the universe that you will have children!

But you know as I do, that waiting is hard. And when it seems to be
going into decades that you're waiting and seeing no fruit of the promise,
you might begin to doubt. Sarah did, wouldn't you at this point?

But the problem isn't that she doubted, the problem is she took that
doubt and tried to take things into her own hands. She decided that Hagar

could provide a son and that would satisfy her and Abraham. But as you can see taking things into our own hands rarely works, as shown in Sarah's story. When we do that, things can go wrong. Why does it happen that way?

Because God has a perfect plan even though it may not seem that way to us right at that moment. Waiting on Him is really the best course of action.

After all, look what happened after Abraham and Sarah truly began to wait on Him. God rewarded their wait and gave them the child He promised them.

Think on These Things

One of the many reasons why it's easy to start taking things into our own hands while we wait is because it's all we seem to be able to think about. Maybe it's time we start thinking on some different things.

Philippians 4:8-9 NIV says:

> *Finally, brothers and sisters, whatever is true, whatever is noble, whatever is right, whatever is pure, whatever is lovely, whatever is admirable—if anything is excellent or praiseworthy—think about such things. Whatever you have learned or received or heard from me, or seen in me—put it into practice. And the God of peace will be with you.*

During our wait, constantly thinking about when the baby will come isn't one of these things that will produce the good things. Because the enemy will come in and create doubt, fear, frustration, anger, etc.

It's time to start thinking about things that are true, noble, right, pure, lovely, admirable, excellent and praiseworthy. Do you know what can fall into these categories? Your husband, your sister, your best friend, your relationship with the Lord, your calling. Start putting your focus onto other things while you wait, things that bring glory and honor to the Lord.

Power Statement

This is a brief statement (similar to an affirmation) that you're setting for yourself of what you will choose to believe about yourself in regards to waiting.

I choose

_____

_____

Questions for discussion:

1. We've all probably heard the story of Abraham and Sarah a thousand times while in the wait. What do you not like or like about their story?
2. Have you ever laughed at something you heard the Lord speak to you? If so, share about that scenario.
3. Have you ever tried to rush the Lord's plan in an area of your life? What led you to do it? What was the outcome?

4

Grief

Grief. When most people hear of the word grief they picture someone who has lost parents or children. But grief can come in all forms, shapes, and sizes. There is no picture perfect look of who deals with grief and what it looks like.

Grief is defined as deep sorrow. What causes deep sorrow? Loss of life (that of a person or pet), loss of a job, loss of a dream, loss of love, friends moving away, the list goes on and on. But the pattern we're seeing is that all sorts of loss cause deep sorrow.

In the world of delayed fertility, we deal with loss of a dream and loss of life. Let's explore these two concepts a bit further:

Loss of a dream—loss of what we thought our family would look like by now. While everyone around us is just having baby after baby, we're watching it happen while it's not happening for us. Each time is just as heart-wrenching as the time before and reminds us of the loss.

Loss of life—loss of the baby growing inside of you before it could even be born. You may try to maintain a pregnancy with no success, and each loss grows a deeper sorrow.

And then there's those things that happen throughout the delayed fertility journey that bring up the sorrow over and over. Birth announcements, baby showers, births, kids starting school, holidays and the list goes on and on. You may feel like everyone wants you to just get over your loss and move forward, but you don't know how and when all these things are brought up time and time again.

1. Your grief is yours and may look different than someone else's.

When you are grieving, don't look at someone else's grief to know what yours should look like. Your grief is different than anyone else's.

It's natural to compare our journey to someone else's journey. Or compare their miracle to our lack of a miracle. You see a friend who just got married become pregnant. And then another one pregnant in less than a year. And then you — it takes years and still nothing. Why her, and why not me? See how we just walked into that comparison trap, we didn't even realize we were doing it, right?

Comparison is a joy killer. Comparing our journey or our grief to someone else's makes us more miserable. It doesn't fix anything. You become bitter and your ability to find happiness for others often become altered. The joy that's taken away takes your eyes away from the One you should be looking at.

> *Dear brothers and sisters, if another believer is overcome by some sin, you who are godly should gently and humbly help that person back onto the right path. And be careful not to fall into the same temptation yourself. Share each other's burdens, and in this way obey the law of Christ. If you think you are too important to help someone, you are only fooling yourself. You are not that important. Pay careful attention to your own work, for then you will get the satisfaction of a job well done, and you won't need to compare yourself to anyone else. For we are each responsible for our own conduct. Those who are taught the word of God should provide for their teachers, sharing all good things with them. Don't be misled—you cannot mock the justice of God. You will always harvest what you plant. Those who live only to satisfy their own sinful nature will harvest decay and death from that sinful nature. But those who live to please the Spirit will harvest everlasting life from the Spirit. So let's*

not get tired of doing what is good. At just the right time we will reap a harvest of blessing if we don't give up. Therefore, whenever we have the opportunity, we should do good to everyone—especially to those in the family of faith.
— Galatians 6:1-10 NLT

You know what, you have enough challenges of your own, why would you look at others and compare yourself to them? You know what else? You don't know what struggles *she* has had. Her struggles are not yours, and yours are not hers. And you know what, your struggles and her struggles all are a part of your individual story. So by comparing yourself to her you're trying to take on her story that was not meant for you. Your story was meant for you. He says you will reap what you sow. If you reap comparison you will sow bitterness, sorrow and a lack of joy.

Your circumstances and your response to them are different than anyone else's. And that is okay.

Give yourself permission to deal with your grief — in your own way and in your own time.

2. You need to process through your grief.

It seems easier to just ignore the grief you feel. Maybe you're tired of grieving. Maybe you're just ready to move forward. But you know what? You can't truly move forward without taking time to grieve. And not just the one time. Each and every time the grief hits you.

Why do you need to acknowledge it each and every time? Because each time that you ignore it, things will start pushing the buttons of that grief. Each time a button gets pressed, it gets bigger and bigger until you completely explode.

That explosion will take someone completely off-guard. You will likely embarrass yourself and you will wish you had handled it differently.

Processing through grief is different for everyone. And there is no right or wrong way to process through your grief.

I was always someone that hated vulnerability and tears. Not only because I didn't want others to see that part of me, but I hated how it made my face feel heavy and it always seemed to bring headaches with the tears. So I avoided dealing with my feelings as much as possible.

So instead of allowing myself to be sad, I became angry. Angry that the thing I wanted most I couldn't have. Angry that my body was failing me. Angry that my spouse and family members didn't understand my anger. Angry that my younger sisters were having babies before I was. And, angry at God because I felt He could change it any moment and He wasn't.

Eventually, my anger caught up with me so much so that tears were the only response I could have. And I swear that I cried and grieved for over a year. I would just bawl and bawl. And I became depressed. I didn't talk to anyone about any of it. I suffered in silence in my grief.

During that year, I had been avoiding church and I worked for my church. I avoided small group, I had avoided talking to people. I had stopped talking and praying to God.

Then God made a way for my husband to send me to an infertility retreat. God met me there. I didn't go looking for Him. I went there for support. I went there to be with other women that understood and what I got was so much greater. My grief was starting to unfold. I was able to share my story and hear others stories, that in itself was so healing. I finally didn't feel alone. For the first time in a long time, I spent time in the Word. And through that time in the Word, He showed me He had never left me. He was always there and the promises He made were still good for me. He showed me that my hope isn't found in the baby or miracle but can only be found in Jesus. And the biggest thing He showed me is that I can have hope because of my security – found in Him. I had been dealing with insecurity, how could I have that hope as long as I was insecure? And how would I be able to fully rest confident in His ability to take care of me and deliver on His promises? I walked away from that event feeling like I had begun processing through my grief.

I look back now and I'm mad at myself for not allowing myself to grieve sooner. Maybe it wouldn't have lasted that long. Maybe I wouldn't have felt so alone for so long. It is what it is now, and I've learned from it.

3. Seek comfort from the ultimate Comforter.

When you first decide that you're ready to process through your grief you may wonder how to do so.

First, allow yourself to cry. Let all of the emotions out, don't hold anything in.

Then, the most important part is allowing God to be your source of comfort.

> *The Lord is close to the brokenhearted and saves those who are crushed in spirit.* — Psalm 34:18 NIV

This scripture tells us that God cares very deeply about our pain. Not only that He cares, but that He wants to reach down and wrap His arms around our hurt and comfort us through it.

I found this to be very true and felt first hand how He longs to rescue me from my pain. I had just found out my sister was pregnant again. I was just broken by it. I was weeping. I didn't want to talk to anyone. And then the Lord led me to this scripture.

So do you know what I did? I spent time in prayer. I told Him how much it hurt. I told Him that it sucked. I told Him that it wasn't fair that my sister got to have another baby while I was still waiting. It was supposed to be my turn. I had some pretty raw emotions, and these were things that in the past I wouldn't have found myself saying to God.

But, I knew that something had to shift; the only way it was going to was if He was true to His word and I allowed Him to demonstrate that in my life. Do you know what happened? I felt so at peace. He truly came in and comforted me like I had never been comforted before. He showed me the "peace that surpasses all understanding" that Philippians 4:7 talked about.

I share this to show you that you can allow Him to comfort you like you've never been comforted before. Allow Him to save you from your grief.

God Hears My Cries & I Can Trust Him

> *Be merciful to me, Lord, for I am in distress; my eyes grow weak with sorrow, my soul and body with grief. My life is consumed by anguish and my years by groaning; my strength fails because of my affliction, and my bones grow weak. ... But I trust in you, Lord; I say, "You are my God." My times are in your*

*hands ... Let your face shine on your servant; save me in your unfailing love.
... How abundant are the good things that you have stored up for those who
fear you, that you bestow in the sight of all, on those who take refuge in you ...
Praise be to the Lord, for he showed me the wonders of his love when I was in
a city under siege. In my alarm I said, "I am cut off from your sight!" Yet you
heard my cry for mercy when I called to you for help. Love the Lord, all his
faithful people! The Lord preserves those who are true to him, but the proud
he pays back in full. Be strong and take heart, all you who hope in the Lord.*
– Psalm 31:9-24 NIV

God is present in our suffering. He can be trusted. His love is unfailing and
he hears our cries for help.

Power Statement

This is a brief statement (similar to an affirmation) that you're setting for
yourself of what you will choose to believe about yourself in regards to grief.

I choose

_____

_____

Questions for discussion:

1. Have you thought of the loss of your dream of having a family as a
   form of grief? Why or why not?
2. Do you tend to look at other people's grief and think theirs is more
   worthy of grieving than yours? Do you still feel that way?
3. Do you tend to spend time allowing yourself to grieve or do you tend
   to try and avoid it? How have you seen this work in your life – has it
   been helpful or hurtful?
4. Have you seen God in the lens of Him caring deeply for your pain
   and hurt? If not, how can you make this shift?

5

Hope and Faith

Grief does this thing where it can totally defeat you. It has the ability to shake everything that is in us. To render us unable to believe in anything good, new or better than what you've currently experienced.

The enemy wants you to sit in your grief and not move from it. Why is that? Because you are not effective when you don't move forward. And maybe your grief will cause you to play the blame game... "Why God? You could change this, why don't you?"

The enemy wants us to blame God because as long as we do, our belief is gone. That's why taking your grief to the Lord is so vital. He has the ability to change things from impossible to possible.

Besides, God may just reveal something to you as you take it to Him; something He's been holding on waiting for you to approach Him.

Turning Grief to Hope

> When hope's dream seems to drag on and on, the delay can be depressing.
> But when at last your dream comes true, life's sweetness will satisfy your soul.
> — Proverbs 13:12 TPT

When days turn into months and months into years, hope is harder and harder to have. Things just look depressing around you.

Maybe like me you've been waiting for years for your family to grow. Each year, you have a little bit of hope that things will change and they don't. So that little bit of hope begins to fade.

I know this was true for me. It's so hard to see the years behind you and believe that things will get better or change.

But then, Scripture goes on to say that what a satisfaction we find when at last our hope becomes a reality.

That right there tells me and it should tell you that that little bit of hope is worth it, even if it doesn't feel like it right now.

Years ago, I was seeking counsel and someone told me sometimes when all you want to do is be angry you just need to put a smile on your face so that eventually that smile will carry itself to the inside. Even though having that little bit of hope will be hard, maybe your face can begin telling your heart and soul to have hope.

> *Return to your fortress, you prisoners of hope; even now I announce that I will restore twice as much to you.* — Zechariah 9:12 NIV

What does it mean to be imprisoned by hope? I believe it means that you are completely sheltered and surrounded by hope. There is no other outcome for you. Hope becomes this thing we have to be in.

We can truly believe God's promise that He will give us two times more and better than what we had before.

More Than

> *Never doubt God's mighty power to work in you and accomplish all this. He will achieve infinitely more than your greatest request, your most unbelievable dream, and exceed your wildest imagination! He will outdo them all, for his miraculous power constantly energizes you.* — Ephesians 3:20 TPT

Do you see that? More than your greatest request and most unbelievable dream? What's your greatest request? Is it to have a baby? He says because of His power that He will exceed that!!! Does that give you something to hope for?

What could "more than you imagine or dream" mean for you? Maybe that means you are not dreaming big enough. How specific are you being in your prayers and requests? I have heard the quote so often that if your dreams don't scare you then they're not going to scare your enemy. Are your dreams big and scary?

If the answer is no, maybe you need to spend some time dreaming and praying. It's time to start believing for bigger and more than you can imagine!

Hope – The Small Feeling

Still unsure about this hope thing? Let's dive into what it really is.

Hope is a feeling that something desired may happen.

So it's just this small feeling that something could happen or change. So imagine that this little feeling of wanting a baby was the thing you were desiring, could be a reality.

This is where we find his strength and comfort, for he empowers us to seize what has already been established ahead of time—an unshakeable hope! We have this certain hope like a strong, unbreakable anchor holding our souls to God himself. – Hebrews 6:18-19 TPT

This small thing is something that God planned for ahead of time – so much so that it's completely unshakeable and unbreakable. Nothing can mess with this small feeling of hope He's given you. He knew you would need this small feeling of hope before you even walked down this road! He was making way for you to have something to believe in.

Are you having a hard time hoping? Pray to Him. Ask Him to give you this unshakeable hope that He already planned for you.

From Him making a way for this hope, to you having this feeling where does this hope go from there?

Now faith brings our hopes into reality and becomes the foundation needed to acquire the things we long for. It is all the evidence required to prove what is still unseen. — Hebrews 11:1 TPT

The Small Feeling Grows

Now our small feeling becomes so unshakeable, where is the only place for it to go? It must develop into faith. Faith is confidence and trust. Faith is a belief that is not based on proof.

This small feeling has become so certain that it has no where else to go then to become a fully confident thing. Even though you have no actual proof of this outcome, it has become so certain that you now trust that this is the reality. This small feeling is not such a small feeling anymore.

My friends, it's time to start grabbing a hold of this small feeling that something can and will change. That this small desire that He's given you to be a mom can happen. Start asking Him to develop this small feeling into the unshakeable hope He started before this would even step into your reality.

Power Statement

This is a brief statement (similar to an affirmation) that you're setting for yourself of what you will choose to believe about yourself in regards to hope and faith.

I choose

_____

_____

Questions for discussion:

1. Have you ever seen God in this light that He has something so much bigger that it topples over anything you've ever thought of? How does this change your perspective?
2. Could you see how God had preplanned an unshakeable hope for you? What would you need to do or believe to capture this unshakeable hope?

3. If you can't have hope for the baby, what is something even smaller that you could have hope for? Maybe it's to make it through today?

4. Can you see your hope becoming so unshakeable that it turns into certainty that you now have this faith — something so strong that you know that this is where He's leading you? If not, what would it take to get you there?

6

Trust & God's Plan

I don't know about you, but when I was in the hardest, deepest pain of my infertility journey, doubt started to creep in. For me, it had nothing to do with who God was because I knew who He was; I just wasn't seeing any evidence of what I thought He had shown me.

I didn't doubt He was a healer; I doubted He would heal *me*.

I didn't doubt He had good plans in store; I doubted He had good plans in store for *me*.

I didn't doubt that He was good; I doubted that He was good to *me*.

I didn't doubt that miracles were possible; I doubted that they would ever be possible for *me*.

Have you ever resonated with that? Have you ever been in a place where you didn't doubt who He was, but that He would ever come through for you? If you were being honest, you saw Him coming through for everyone else but you. Yep, that's what was going on with me.

For me, it took a very long time for it to even get to that place. When I really look at it, it wasn't doubt, but rather a lack of trust of God. It made me question if I really believed if He was true to His word.

Maybe like me you have felt this too, and maybe like me you don't want to admit it to yourself. I didn't want to put out there that I didn't trust God because I was raised to never doubt or question God. I mean He's God! He created the universe, so who am I to doubt Him? This school of thought caused me to deal with some heavy things internally that I never wanted to bring out, and it just continued to keep me held down, quiet and completely alone.

It took a long time to realize that God could handle everything I have inside of me. He created me, so nothing I could say or do could surprise Him. He knows me intricately, every piece of me. It took hearing it from another author and from a Pastor saying the same thing to me. Even after hearing that from them, I still struggled to really say how I was feeling. I was afraid; what if He didn't love me the same or what if He disowned me?

How could I think the God of everlasting love, a God that loves me so completely that He forgave every sin I ever committed, the God of that Romans 8:38-39 kind of love could ever stop loving me or disown me?

After all, it says:

> ... neither death nor life, neither angels nor demons, neither the present nor the future, nor any powers, neither height nor depth, nor anything else in all creation, will be able to separate us from the love of God that is in Christ Jesus our Lord. —Romans 8:38-39 NIV

The God we serve, could never ever ever stop loving us. Love is who He is.

> Whoever does not love does not know God, because God is love. —1 John 4:8 NIV

So that means I was able to be honest with myself and with God. And you can, too. If you're feeling like you can't trust Him, I get it. God can handle it. Honestly, I wish I would have been brave enough to bring it straight to God, but that's not what happened for me. I hid from it for so long that God confronted me with it. Ha! Sometimes, you don't really want Him to have to confront you with it, but like we just talked about, He's a loving God.

Why Trust Him?

Before we can find out why we should trust Him, let's look at what trust is. Trust is: a firm belief in the reliability, truth, ability, or strength of someone or something. So when we trust God, we are saying we believe that He is true to His word and that He is strong enough to do what He said He will do.

So, what does God's Word have to say about trust?

1. When I trust in Him, He will never forsake me.

> *Those who know your name trust in you, for you, Lord, have never forsaken those who seek you.* —Psalm 9:10 NIV

I can trust in God because he will never leave me or give up on me. When I seek Him, know Him, and follow Him, He is always by my side. When fear starts to creep in, all I have to do is seek Him and I'll see that He hasn't left me at all.

2. When I trust in Him, I will see a reward.

> *Commit your way to the Lord; trust in him and he will do this: He will make your righteous reward shine like the dawn ...* — Psalm 37:5-6 NIV

When we trust Him, He will make our reward shine like the dawn. But what does that even mean? Well, let's look at this for a moment. What do you think of when you think of the dawn or morning? I think of a new day coming. I think of "beautiful" and I think of "bright". When I look at this Scripture in this context, it's saying my reward will be new, beautiful and bright. Something I've never seen or experienced in my life, something that is so beautiful that it can only come from God, and so bright that it radiates from Him.

3. When I trust in Him, He directs me.

> *Let the morning bring me word of your unfailing love, for I have put my trust in you. Show me the way I should go, for to you I entrust my life.* — Psalm 143:8 NIV

Trust in the Lord with all your heart and lean not on your own understanding; in all your ways submit to him, and he will direct your paths. — Proverbs 3:5-6 NIV

Do you ever struggle with what direction to go next or what steps you should take? That's the beauty of trusting God, He already has our steps mapped out and the plan for our life. All we have to do is place our trust in Him and He will direct us. Unsure on where He's directing you? Prayer is a big piece of this puzzle as well.

The big doozie here in Proverbs 3:5-6 is not leaning on our own understanding. That means that if we are expecting Him to direct us and if we are putting our complete trust in Him, we have to let go of the control. We have to try to not map out our own steps. We have to put it completely in His hands and truly surrender.

4. When I trust in Him, He gives me peace.

You will keep in perfect peace those whose minds are steadfast, because they trust in you. —Isaiah 26:3 NIV

Peace? Can I even experience it? The answer is yes! God says when we trust in Him completely with unwavering trust, He will keep us in peace. In order to keep us in peace, He had to give us peace to begin with. Do you need some peace — in your mind, heart, emotions? Trust Him completely. You know what you'll experience? That Philippians 4:7 kind of peace.

Trusting in God's Plan

One of the biggest steps in trusting God is trusting wholeheartedly in His plans for our life. Even when things don't make sense to us — when things don't look the way we anticipated. That's hard, right?!?!

I want to share something that was hugely revolutionary for me in really beginning to trust His plan for my life regarding my fertility and future family.

A friend shared with me that we often spend time thinking and praying about how we want a child and how we want him or her in our own time. But, the kicker is this, have we ever taken the time to think about the perfect time for that child to be born? Wait... what?!?!

Well, let's look at what Scripture says. Ecclesiastes 3:1-2 NIV says, *"There is a time for everything, and a season for every activity under the heavens: a time to be born ..."* So that means, there is a perfect time for your child to be born. Why does it have to be the right time? Does your child need to marry someone that they'll meet at a specific point in their life? Does your child have a specific calling on their life that has to happen at a certain age and time? Or, maybe one of the generations after your child will be impacted by when your child is born.

Let's take a look at the genealogy of Joseph.

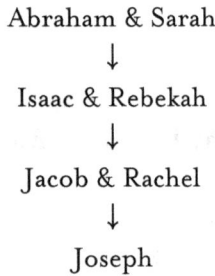

Abraham & Sarah

↓

Isaac & Rebekah

↓

Jacob & Rachel

↓

Joseph

Do you see that? Joseph comes directly from Abraham. And do you see who comes from Abraham? It's Isaac! Just about everyone that has struggled with their fertility journey knows that Abraham & Sarah dealt with barrenness. God had promised them a child. But it took a long time for Him to deliver their son, over 100 years!!!

Now let's think about this. Do you think that if Isaac was born right when Abraham and Sarah wanted him that all the plans and callings God had for all of their descendants would be fulfilled?

Absolutely not! If Isaac was born on their time table, then Joseph wouldn't have been able to save His family at the time he was needed to save them. Because Joseph would have been born at least 75 years sooner than God planned. I don't know about you, but that's mind-blowing to me.

So what can we learn from this? We can learn that just because we think it's the right time, doesn't mean that it actually is. God sees everything in our future and our children's future and their children's future. So He knows the right time for our children. God's plan for our fertility journey is a perfect plan that we can have complete trust in. We may not see in front of us what the reasons are, but He has the full picture so we need to trust Him.

Power Statement

This is a brief statement (similar to an affirmation) that you're setting for yourself of what you will choose to believe about yourself in regards to trust and God's plan.

I choose

_____

_____

Questions for discussion:

1. Seeking Him directly relates to Him being by our side, and gives us the ability to trust Him. How have you been doing at seeking Him? Is there something you need to work on to seek Him more?
2. Do you tend to lean towards your own understanding or waiting on His direction? Why or why not?
3. What does peace mean to you?
4. Have you ever thought about there being a perfect time for your child to be born? How might this change your perception of your fertility journey?

7

The Struggle of Prayer

Prayer. Such a vital piece of our relationship with God. But, it may be one of the hardest things to take part in when dealing with delayed fertility or any major struggle. Is praying hard for you during the season you're in? I know it's been hard for me.

Why is prayer a struggle on this journey? Maybe you've been angry. Maybe you've been doubting God. Maybe you've been feeling very distant. And, maybe just maybe, with how you're feeling the last thing you want to do is talk to God.

I struggled with knowing He could change my circumstances at any moment, and He chose not to. So that made me not want to approach prayer and conversation with Him. And, like I talked about in the last chapter, I also wasn't sure that if I decided to finally talk I was ready to share how I was really feeling.

Knowing God could heal me at any moment, knowing He could miraculously fill my womb and knowing He could give me all the answers I was searching for and then knowing He wasn't doing that — it completely wrecked me. It had me on the floor in my closet in tears. It had me unable to breathe. It had me in a place of doubting everything He had been telling me about my future. How was my God who loves me unconditionally not delivering immediately when I knew He could? I didn't understand why. *(Side note: the answer I found to why He wasn't delivering when I knew He could can be found in the last chapter where I talked about God's plan.)*

Does any of this sound like some of the reasons you haven't wanted to pray? I completely understand, so believe me, there's no judgment here. I was in your shoes. Like I said, it took God chasing me down and making me listen to Him.

Now that we've talked about why you might not want to pray, let's talk about why you might.

Why pray?

Prayer is so important. There are so many reasons to pray. You may need time to mourn or just be, I get it. But let's not leave things there. Prayer has to be introduced into your life and here are some of the reasons why.

1. Praying builds our relationship with God.

Have you ever gone any length of time not talking to a friend? Maybe several months or years? This likely created a distance between you. You weren't close. I mean, how could you be? If you're not pouring into your relationship, it will go stagnant.

The same is true with our relationship with God. If we don't spend time talking to Him in prayer, our relationship goes stagnant. We can't truly get to know Him better, understand Him, build on our love for Him or know His heart unless we're talking to Him. When we talk to Him, our lives are better for it and we get closer to Him, which forms a deeper intimacy with Him.

It's amazing how we'll begin to see how much He truly loves us when we spend time with Him.

2. God hears us when we pray and answers us.

> This is the confidence we have in approaching God: that if we ask anything according to his will, he hears us. — 1 John 5:14 NIV

If you believe, you will receive whatever you ask for in prayer.
— Matthew 21:22 NIV

Therefore I tell you, whatever you ask for in prayer, believe that you have received it, and it will be yours. — Mark 11:24 NIV

To me, it's so comforting to know that when I spend time talking with God I'm not wasting my time, but He's actively listening to me. I can be sure that He will listen to every word I speak, and my prayers are not falling on deaf ears.

The caveat to having deep communication with God is that we have to believe and we have to ask anything according to His will. How do you know if it's in line with His will? Check what the Word says about it. If you don't see it in the Word, ask Him if it's in His will and He will direct you.

3. To bring your prayer requests to Him and leave them with Him.

And pray in the Spirit on all occasions with all kinds of prayers and requests.
— Ephesians 6:18a NIV

Do not be anxious about anything, but in every situation, by prayer and petition, with thanksgiving, present your requests to God.
— Philippians 4:6 NIV

Praying about your requests I believe is two-folded. Even though God knows our needs and our requests before we bring them before Him, I believe He wants to hear about them from us as it builds relationship with Him, it allows Him the opportunity to connect with us and it demonstrates to Him that we love Him by inviting Him into our lives. Praying about your requests is also a way for you to release your needs to God and take your worry and anxiety away. This demonstrates to God your faith in Him, in His ability, power and overall belief in His desire to be good to you. It shows Him that you believe that nothing is too big for God, that your present circumstances do not limit Him in any way and that you can seek His help and comfort to make it through what's currently in front of you. This takes things out of your hands and puts them in God's hands. We don't want to do what Sarah did and start taking them into our own hands.

And the last benefit about praying about your requests comes in the next verse…

4. He brings a peace that can't be explained.

And the peace of God, which transcends all understanding, will guard your hearts and your minds in Christ Jesus. — Philippians 4:7 NIV

You might be sensing a theme here since this isn't the first time I've mentioned this scripture. Growing up, anytime my dad heard me worrying about something, he would say "Philippians 4:6 & 7". I mean all the time, several times a week as a teenager. After hearing me bring up this scripture a few times, you may start to understand my annoyance with my dad, ha! He used to beat me up with Philippians 4:6-7 every time he heard me getting anxious about anything.

But in all seriousness, this verse is one of my favorites. He's telling us that when we bring our requests to Him and leave them at His feet, He's going to provide a peace like nothing we've ever experienced and it can't be explained. This peace will begin to change our hearts and minds because we are so much at peace.

I was dealing with some heavy anxiety and fear over an important meeting I had to go into that could directly affect our path to becoming parents. My stomach hurt so bad I thought I was going to throw up. I was putting myself through turmoil over it. And all of a sudden God brought to my remembrance the scripture Philippians 4:6-7. So I started praying and asking Him to give me peace that passes all understanding, to calm my nerves, grant us favor, give us words to speak, calm my anxiety about all the unknowns. It was then that I experienced this kind of peace myself that we're talking about — it was as if I didn't have a care in the world, like I had never been worried, panicked or been afraid — it was as if the ocean had just run over my anxiety like it does with the sand, covering it and bringing a calmness. I knew I didn't have to worry about it anymore, because He had it covered. The peace I felt didn't make sense at all. I mean, I should've panicked – butterflies in my stomach, heart racing, mind filling with fearful thoughts – as that's normally what would happen for me. But, in all honesty should we really be panicked if the God who made the universe, the God that crafted the galaxies – has it all in His hands and mapped out? Did you know that the sun is 92,000 miles from earth and if you got close you would burn up? These are the kind of details God orchestrated. So believe me, He definitely can handle every detail you bring Him.

5. He will not hold your prayer against you.

> He will respond to the prayer of the destitute; he will not despise their plea.
> – Psalm 102:17 NIV

After talking about this some in the last chapter, I'm not sure about you, but seeing it in the Scripture so plainly gave me so much relief and confidence in approaching Him with everything – not just the easy things, but the hard things, too.

I realized how not talking to Him about everything was holding me back. It was like keeping me in this prison, because these things were building up in me and only hurting me. It's like when you haven't told someone in your personal life something you've needed to tell them for so long because you're afraid of how they'll react or you don't like dealing with the conflict of it – once you finally do, there's just such a relief and peace that comes over you because it's finally out there. And after you've been able to work through that thing, it just develops a sweetness between you – you deal with the elephant in the room and it brings you even closer.

That's what having the freedom to tell God everything – the easy and hard things – does. It brings you so much closer to Him. You've revealed part of your heart and your pain and now He can truly help you process through it; there's no mountain standing in between you and Him. You've removed it, so now you are so much closer to Him. As you continue to do this, the love and trust you've needed to develop with Him will also continue to form. This is what it's all about!

6. Jesus intercedes for us.

> *My prayer is not for them alone. I pray also for those who will believe in me through their message...* — John 17:20 NIV

Jesus is praying for you to Father God on your behalf! Why would He do that? Because He loves us! He cares deeply about you!

He continues in that passage to say that He desires for us to be in Him and Father God so that they may believe in Him and so that others can see God's glory! You should really go read John 17:20-26. It's so good!

Jesus desires for His glory to be revealed through us. Could that mean that your fertility story is being developed so that others may see God's glory and believe in Him because of what they've seen Him do in your life? I fully believe in this! Our Father loves to give good gifts especially so He can demonstrate His love through us to reach His other children.

7. The Bible says to persistently pray.

> *Be joyful in hope, patient in affliction, faithful in prayer.* — Romans 12:12 NIV

> *Rejoice always, pray continually, give thanks in all circumstances; for this is God's will for you in Christ Jesus.* — 1 Thessalonians 5:16-18 NIV

Here we are told to faithfully pray continually. The interesting thing here is it's also talking about rejoicing in both scriptures. I believe that when we learn to be joyful, it will give us a desire to pray continually. We'll want to be connected with Him on the regular.

How do we tap into this joy when we're dealing with struggle and grief? Nehemiah 8:10 says, *"Do not grieve, for the joy of the Lord is your strength."* Here, we find that our true strength lies in the joy of the Lord. That means we find joy in Him!

8. Prayer is effective and brings healing.

Is anyone among you in trouble? Let them pray. Is anyone happy? Let them sing songs of praise. Is anyone among you sick? Let them call the elders of the church to pray over them and anoint them with oil in the name of the Lord. And the prayer offered in faith will make the sick person well; the Lord will raise them up. If they have sinned, they will be forgiven.
–James 5:13-15 NIV

Prayer is healing in so many ways. Healing for the sick, healing for your sin. Healing for your heart. God is a healer and He uses prayer to heal us!

Some prayer will require you to have leaders pray over you! After all, in Matthew 18:20 NIV Jesus says, *"For where two or three gather in my name, there am I with them."* The above scripture from James talks about leaders anointing with oil. If you haven't done this for your fertility journey, I highly recommend it.

Some instances will require fasting and prayer. Isaiah 58:6 & 8 NIV says, *"Is not this the kind of fasting I have chosen: to loose the chains of injustice and untie the cords of the yoke, to set the oppressed free and break every yoke?... Then your light will break forth like the dawn, and your healing will quickly appear; then your righteousness will go before you, and the glory of the Lord will be your rear guard."*

9. When couples prayed for children, He answered.

Isaac prayed to the Lord on behalf of his wife, because she was childless. The Lord answered his prayer, and his wife Rebekah became pregnant.
— Genesis 25:21 NIV

And by faith even Sarah, who was past childbearing age, was enabled to bear children because she considered him faithful who had made the promise.
— Hebrews 11:11 NIV

But the angel said to him: "Do not be afraid, Zechariah; your prayer has been heard. Your wife Elizabeth will bear you a son, and you are to call him John."
— Luke 1:13 NIV

These are just a few examples of the couples God rewarded with children when they prayed and asked. This gives me so much hope, and I hope it does the same for you.

I want to add a disclaimer that there is an example of someone in the Bible that didn't have a child, Michal, David's wife. Beth Forbus of Sarah's Laughter shared with me her thoughts on Michal. She says "Most theologians and historians do not actually believe Michal was barren but that the reason for her childlessness was a breakdown in the relationship with David due to her ridiculing him when he worshipped God so profoundly. I tend to believe this because of a couple of different reasons. Because of how she publicly ridiculed the king their relationship most likely was never the same again. According to tradition, he would have had her banished to another part of the palace. They very possibly could have lived the rest of their lives without ever seeing each other again, much less ever having a sexual relationship again. I also tend to believe this because Scripture actually calls every barren woman barren. It doesn't call her barren. It says she had no children until the day of her death."

I don't know the reasons why some women never have children, only God has those answers. What I do know is that of the six women mentioned in the Bible that were barren, they all eventually had children. So, if God has placed the desire in your heart to have children, keep the faith, keep praying. He desires to give good gifts to you!

Power Statement
This is a brief statement (similar to an affirmation) that you're setting for yourself of why you will choose to pray.

I choose

_____

_____

Questions for discussion:

1. Have you ever been scared to tell God how you truly felt? What were your fears? What truths from God's word can you replace those feelings/fears with? How can you take a step forward in speaking honestly with God?

2. Do you have a story of healing that came through prayer? Share about it!

3. Is there someone in your life who's dealt with infertility and been able to start their family that has encouraged you? Share with us so we can be encouraged as well.

4. How can you begin to open your heart back up to prayer and what steps will you take?

8

The Vision of Marriage

I think most of us had those little girl dreams about marriage and their wedding day. We all watched the fairy tale movies that get us all excited about our fairy tale ending of meeting the perfect guy. We'll have a beautiful wedding, an amazing marriage, have babies and of course, the house with a white picket fence!

Things rarely turn out the way you expect. There's so much energy spent on making your wedding day fabulous, most of us don't actually prepare or invest time into preparing for the actual marriage. Some couples do the best they can and do premarital counseling, but not everyone does.

No one really talks about the problems you will run into: financial problems, communication issues, jobs, moves, etc. Then there are those of us that deal with adultery or infertility. How do you handle these things when you didn't prepare for them? It's definitely not easy! It takes a lot of compromise and constantly dying to yourself! And I don't know of people who actually prepare couples for the prospect that having a child may be very difficult for 1 in 8 couples.

Maybe the beginning of your marriage was a little rocky as you navigated the new married couple waters, but you eventually figured it out, as most of us do. That doesn't mean you don't run into problems.

But what do you do when after trying for quite a while, you both are faced with the reality that getting pregnant doesn't come easily for you? What happens when you're now at doctors appointments faced with decisions about treatments or you now have to discuss the possibility of foster care or adoption? Those decisions are hard, but even harder when you didn't have a plan before you got married. As we know, tests and treatments and adoption are not cheap. And most of us don't have insurance or government support that will cover the cost. So, now you're faced with more financial challenges – figuring out how will you determine if you'll proceed with treatments or adoption and if you can even afford it.

At this point, you might be fighting about what to do next and it could create a rift between the two of you. Especially if one of you wants to go one direction and the other one wants to go a different direction. How do you navigate these big decisions when you're not on the same page?

On top of that, infertility can start to affect your sex life and sex becomes technical. It's all about getting pregnant now. With your intimacy being affected, neither one of you feels desirable and this can make you feel distant from the person you're sharing your life with.

Marriage was not designed to be this way. Genesis 2:22-24 NIV says, *"Then the Lord God made a woman from the rib he had taken out of the man, and he brought her to the man. The man said, "This is now bone of my bones and flesh of my flesh; she shall be called 'woman,' for she was taken out of man." That is why a man leaves his father and mother and is united to his wife, and they become one flesh."* You see, we were meant to be one – to cooperate together as one body. In verse 18 it even says *"It is not good for the man to be alone. I will make a helper suitable for him."* The wives in the marriage relationship were created to complement their husbands, to be their helpmate.

But how do we get back to the way marriage was designed? How do we complement each other and be each other's helpmate?

Getting Back to One

It's time we implement some safeguards in our marriage so that we can truly bring marriage back to its original design.

First, we have to make our marriage a priority. Next to our relationship to God, it has got to be our top priority. That means <u>more important than having a child</u>. More important than your job. Your spouse needs to be your priority.

Ways to make it a priority:

- **Spend time praying together every morning or night.** The best way you can build your relationship is to seek God and get closer to the Lord. The closer you are to the Lord as a couple, the closer you'll be as a couple.
- **Talk throughout the day.** Write each other notes, text each other, talk on the phone. Don't just limit your conversations to when you get home for the day. When you talk to each other consider complementing each other. Find things you love about them and make sure they know.
- **Take regular date nights.** There are things you can do that don't cost anything or you can be more elaborate. Picnics, concerts, attending church events, marriage conferences, dinner and a movie, working out together, museums, mini road trips, karaoke, dancing, game night, bowling, going to an escape room, binge watching a show on Netflix and so much more. Just get creative with it.
- **Keep sex in your marriage for intimacy.** Yes, there are times where it has to be about building your family. But you have to be intentional to bring sex into your marriage for the purpose of intimacy. Discuss this together and decide what that looks like for you as a couple.

Next, how you deal with disagreements is very important. You have to determine how you will handle it when as a couple you don't agree on something. Determine the level of disagreement. Is this a code orange – a mild disagreement, but something you could discuss if you had a little space ? Or, is this a code red – as in, you just might strangle them if they keep talking or you don't know if you'll ever come to an agreement about this one?

If it's code orange, then agree to give each other some space to think things over and come back to it in a few hours. There is no reason to make this issue turn into a code red. If you still can't come to an agreement, it's time for both of you separately to pray about it. I think after some time in prayer, you'll know what to do to resolve it.

If it's code red, there's a couple things you can do here. Definitely don't talk about it until everyone is calm. If after talking about it, you still can't resolve it, it's time to determine a few things. Is this a very bad fight, and not about making a decision? Maybe you need to bring in a neutral party or maybe it will even need some counsel to resolve. If it's about making a big decision that you can't agree on, I've found the best thing is to pray about it and not approach it with my spouse until God speaks to my spouse or I on what we're supposed to do. Again, this also may take some counsel. The biggest thing we have to realize is that we can't always resolve things right away, and that's okay. And we have to realize it's okay to bring a counselor or neutral party to help us determine the best course of action.

There are many times I've heard from the Lord on something and I know my husband isn't quite there yet. So I've had to pray about it for a while, and just ask God to speak to my husband's heart. Eventually, he came around. Because in the end, God's plan will prevail. And sometimes it's been the other way around.

We have to remember our spouse is not our enemy.

> *The thief comes only to steal and kill and destroy; I have come that they may have life, and have it to the full.* — John 10: 10 NIV

> *For our struggle is not against flesh and blood, but against the rulers, against the authorities, against the powers of this dark world and against the spiritual forces of evil in the heavenly realms.* — Ephesians 6:12 NIV

> *Be alert and of sober mind. Your enemy the devil prowls around like a roaring lion looking for someone to devour.* — 1 Peter 5:8 NIV

We have a real enemy and it's time we recognize when he's messing with our marriage. The enemy doesn't want our marriage to succeed. He wants division and failed marriages. He doesn't want our purpose as a couple to prevail. We have to begin to pray against the enemy, and declaring that he can't have our marriage and that our marriage is protected and belongs to God.

That brings up my last tip for keeping the oneness in your relationship. We have to develop our vision for our marriage — *Write the vision; make it plain on tablets, so he may run who reads it.* (Habakkuk 2:2 ESV)

We have to know our general vision for our marriage and each year what our vision is that year. Jimmie Evans has this book, *Mountaintop of Marriage: A Vision Retreat Guidebook*, where you actually go on a retreat together and develop your vision. One of the biggest things the author stresses is the importance to get away to develop your vision, as life comes with so many distractions, and you need to be able to spend devoted time on this. My husband and I love this guidebook as it really walks you through the entire process of establishing your vision, from your overall vision for your marriage, to having one for your family traditions and even the values and vision for your children. It also walks you through setting goals for different areas like finances, your spiritual lives, sexual lives and more. To top it all off, it helps you set milestones and the vision for your marriage for the next 12 months. Through this book, we were able to establish that our marriage exists to be each other's helpmate through our lives, while growing and strengthening each other as we model Christ's love to each other. We feel this book offers so much value for our marriage, so we encourage you to check it out as well.

Ultimately, it all comes back to remembering that we are one, not against each other.

Power Statement

This is a brief statement (similar to an affirmation) that you're setting for yourself of what you will choose for your marriage.

I choose

_____

_____

Questions for discussion:

1. What are the biggest challenges you've faced in your marriage?
2. What can you do to make your marriage a priority?
3. Do you have any examples of having to give time to cool off or pray and then see your spouse's mind changed? Share about that experience.
4. Do you have a challenge recognizing that your spouse is not your enemy? How can you renew your mind and see them differently?

9

Find the Good

In closing, we have to talk about how to find the good in this journey to motherhood or fatherhood. When you deal with disappointments, losses and fertility delay, finding the good is so very hard.

A pregnancy test is negative. A treatment fails. A birth mom changes her mind. You lose the baby. Let's be honest, there's not much, if any good to be found in these things.

The biggest good I have seen is realizing there is a perfect time for everything and that includes the birth of your child.

The pregnancy test might be negative or the treatment might fail because your son isn't supposed to be born for another year. Maybe God has something to teach you or maybe there's something specific your son needs to do at a specific time, which means he can't be born now.

The birth mom changing her mind for the adoption might be happening because that child is not the child God designed to be raised by you and your spouse. Maybe He has so much better for you, for your future child and for the birth mom.

I honestly don't know what good if any could come from losing a child. It's ugly. It's horrible. And, it just plain sucks. If no one has said this to you, I want you to hear/read me saying this - I am so sorry for your loss. I'm sorry that that little life never got to be on the outside with you. I'm sorry you missed out on life with them, and I'm sorry their life was cut too short. I'm sorry for all the things people have said to you trying to help but only making it worse. I'm sorry that people might act like your loss doesn't matter or that they weren't a real part of your life. Loss and death is awful no matter what side of things it happens. Your loss matters. Your child mattered to you and to God and to others around you. Your grief matters.

Friends, we have to begin to reach into each other's world and educate ourselves. I'm tired of people not understanding what's going on and saying or doing something hurtful. Let's be the change we want to see in our own lives. Start asking questions when someone is going through something that you don't understand. Saying something like, "I'm sorry that you're going through this. I absolutely have no idea what that's like. Could you explain to me what it's like for you? Can you tell me how I can support you?" would show the kind of support that person truly needs.

Regardless if there is good in each of those things, there is still good to be found in your life. It doesn't have to be found in your fertility journey. I heard someone say "every day may not be good, but there is good in every day". It's time to discover things that are good in your life.

Here are some goods to be found in our fertility journey:

- New sisters/friends you've made in the infertility community
- Discovering your true strength
- Learning how to really be a listener for your friends
- Finding the value in educating yourself in serious things
- Doing something you might not have never done without delayed fertility

What are some good things to be found in our life:

- Nieces & nephews
- Furbabies

- A job that provides for your family
- Your spouse
- God
- Vacation/traveling
- Hobbies
- Sunset
- Movies
- Church
- Small Groups

I want to implore you to wake up every day and choose to find the good. Determine that in the midst of everything you have been through (or are currently going through) to find the good.

When you begin to change the words you use about your fertility journey, wait well, process through your grief, have hope and faith for your journey and in God, trust God and accept His plan for your life, embrace a lifestyle of prayer, unite as one with your spouse making your marriage a priority and find the good in the journey you will be at the sweet place of being able to bravely embrace your infertility journey with dignity and grace. You'll truly be embracing bravery in Him. I am so confident in you and your ability to do all these things through Him who strengthens you. I'm believing with you!

Power Statement
This is a brief statement (similar to an affirmation) that you're setting for yourself of what/why you're choosing to find the good in.

I choose

_____

_____

Questions for discussion:

1. Is finding the good a hard thing for you to grasp? Why or why not?

2. How can you begin to educate others on what delayed fertility and/or loss is like and how they can support you?

3. Maybe it's from the list or maybe it's not, what is one thing you can find the good in your fertility journey?

4. How can you make finding the good a daily occurrence for you?

Appendix A

FOR SUPPORT GROUP LEADERS / FACILITATORS

I wrote this book specifically for you, the support group leader. Doing support groups through Embrace Bravery has made me very passionate about having material to use in support group. That's why I wrote this with support groups in mind. I want you to be able to use this book in your groups and walk people through the content. So below I will provide you a few tips on how to best use the material.

1. I suggest you read through the material yourself prior to using this in the group. You need to be as familiar with this content as possible. Go through this book for yourself, meaning walk through it all, read it, answer the questions for yourself. Experience it personally. This will help you walk others through the material.

2. If you haven't led a support group, yet, then this tip is for you: For your first group meeting, do a few icebreaker questions (google small group icebreaker questions, there are so many great ideas out there). This will help you all get to know each other a little and help with anyone that might be nervous about talking. You should spend most of your first meeting sharing your fertility stories/journey's. You will want to get to know each other and know what each of you are walking through.

3. Also at the first meeting, make sure everyone has gotten the *Embrace Bravery* book, and ask them to read the introduction and

chapter 1 prior to the next group meeting. If you have already been meeting with this group previously, communicate this same thing prior to launching the study. You'll want everyone coming prepared having read the material. Encourage them that as they read the material to highlight anything that sticks out to them and underline anything that is challenging. Also, explain the power statement, how it works and that they should do that on their own time, as this needs to be a personal thing they're choosing to affirm in their lives.

4. When you gather to dive into the book, start off your meetings with prayer. Invite the Lord into your time together. Ask Him to speak through you and to lead the group's discussion. Pray that He reveals anything He wants your group to get out of the material to come forth. And pray for the women that are there that their hearts would be encouraged as you talk through the content.

5. Following prayer, start off the discussion by asking anyone to share the things they highlighted or underlined. What stood out to each of you from this chapter? Was there anything that was challenging for you? Let's talk about those things first.

6. Ask each of the group discussion questions from the end of the chapter. Give plenty of time for people to answer. If it's quiet, don't immediately move on. Sometimes people just need some time to be brave enough to speak. And sometimes they're waiting for someone else to go first. In most cases, you should be the last one to share. Unless, after waiting some time and no one answers, then you might want to break the ice and answer. A lot of times this will open the floor and others will share.

7. If after you've gone through all the questions, you still have more time left, I'm providing additional questions for each chapter below. Feel free to use these in group if time allows. But, make sure you leave space for prayer at the end of the meeting.

8. Pray. Ask for prayer requests. It could be specific to their fertility journey or it could be related to the material. But you need to pray for each other. This will strengthen your bond as a group, and will

allow you to apply what you're learning. Each group meeting, you should follow up on the prayer requests from the previous meeting and ask how things are going related to the previous requests. If they received an answer to their prayer and it was positive, take time to celebrate the praise reports. If things have gotten harder, mourn with them, relate to them. Make sure they know you care about what they're going through. And keep praying about these things they're requesting.

9. All in all, I want you to use this material to help each of you grow in your fertility journey. You are together to learn how to embrace your fertility story with dignity and strength. You are there together to learn how to support each other. You are there together so each of you knows you are not alone in this. Allow this material to help you do this. If you need to change something to work differently for your group, then do it. Always do what is best for your group.

I'm praying with you that this material will be an amazing experience for you and your group!

Embracing bravery together,

Shannon

Additional Questions for Discussion:

Chapter 1

1. What scripture can you begin to speak over yourself in regards to feeling broken?
2. What scripture can you begin to speak over yourself in regards to being worthy for motherhood?
3. Do you tend to be a negative Nancy with your words?
4. Do you see the value in the thoughts and words you speak being more positive?
5. Read Psalm 113:9. What does it say you will be?
6. What has been the source of your identity?
7. Of the descriptions of what God says you are, which one speaks to you the most? Why?

Chapter 2

1. Who do you consider brave and why?
2. What's the most important quality to qualify someone as brave?
3. What makes you feel weak? Why?
4. What is something you've stepped out in despite your fear?
5. Did you ever start to doubt after you stepped out?
6. What can you begin to do bravely in your fertility journey?

Chapter 3

1. What comes to mind when you think of waiting?
2. What are some other areas you tend to be waiting on/in?
3. Have you questioned the purpose for waiting? What have you considered was the purpose?
4. Have you ever thought of God working on your behalf behind the scenes? How does it make you feel? What are some areas that you now realize He might have been working behind the scenes?
5. When you have felt worn down by your wait, have you found yourself going to God to strengthen you? Why or why not?
6. If you've relied on God's strength, what were the results?
7. Have you sensed God's protection? What does God's help look like for you in your wait?
8. Have you felt like you could wait expectantly? What has held you back if you haven't felt that way? If you have felt that way, what led you there and what have been the results?
9. Why do you think it's important to wait on the Lord?
10. What things can you begin thinking on while in your wait?

Chapter 4

1. What types of grief have you been dealing with?
2. Do you seek comfort from the Ultimate Comforter easily? Why or why not?
3. If seeking comfort from God is hard for you, why?
4. What does peace that surpasses all understanding look like to you?

Chapter 5

1. Do you tend to stay in the camp of grief? How do you pull yourself out once you've processed through the pain?
2. Do you find it challenging to have hope for something better? What would it take to start believing?

3. What is the hope for you? What is the small feeling you could believe for?

Chapter 6

1. Do you struggle with trusting God? Why or why not?
2. If you've dealt with doubting God, share your story — what led to it and how you learned to silence the doubt and trust God.
3. What does complete trust look like to you?
4. In regards to fertility, did you ever feel like He had forsaken or abandoned you? How can you take your feelings and turn them to trust?
5. When I trust Him I will see a new reward. While this is not the reason to trust Him, it's definitely a benefit of trusting HIm. What kind of new reward do you think you might see from Him?
6. What other benefits do you think come from trusting Him?
7. How have you dealt with feeling like you don't know which direction to go?
8. How can you begin to fully trust God's plan for your fertility journey?

Chapter 7

1. What is your prayer life like right now?
2. Are you now or have you ever avoided prayer? If so, what reasons were/are you avoiding it?
3. Has prayer built your relationship with the Lord? Share about this experience.
4. Why do you think prayer is important?
5. Did you know Jesus intercedes/prays for you? What feelings does that produce in you?
6. God hears us and answers us. Sometimes the answer is yes, and sometimes it is no. Like a parent, his no is usually to protect us. Have you experienced his no answer? Share about it.
7. How often do you spend time in prayer? If you haven't been praying

lately, when you were praying how much time were you spending? If it's not much time, what can you do to increase the time you spend in prayer?

8. Where do you find you have the most focused prayer? Is it in a prayer/war room? A shower? Your room? A closet? If you don't have a place, maybe it's time to have a place devoted to prayer. Where could this space be? What could you have in this space?

Chapter 8

1. What was your impression of what marriage would be like before you got married? Has it lived up to your expectations?
2. Were you focused on the wedding day more than the marriage? What can you do now to be focused on your marriage?
3. Is your marriage a priority? Why or why not?
4. How often are your date nights?
5. Are there some date night ideas you'd like to try out?
6. Are your disagreements more code orange or code red? Are there any tips from this chapter that could help you learn to recognize the level and how to move forward?
7. Do you create visions for your marriage? If not, would you consider doing a vision retreat? Why or why not?

Chapter 9

1. If you've had negative pregnancy tests or failed treatments, could you see what good you could find in that? Share about that.
2. If you've had an adoption fall through, could you see what good you could find in that? Share about that experience.
3. If you've had a loss of a child, what is something you want other people to know about it {what it's like for you, how people can help, etc.}?
4. Maybe it's from the list or maybe it's not, what is one thing you can find the good in your life?

Appendix B

RESOURCES

Download your Power Statement Graphic Template to your phone to create your own Power Statement Graphics!

1. Dr. Caroline Leaf: https://drleaf.com/about/toxic-thoughts/
2. Bible.org: https://bible.org/article/who-does-god-say-i-am
3. Christianity Today: https://www.christianitytoday.com/iyf/faithandlife/devotionals/what-does-bible-say-about-me.html

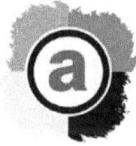
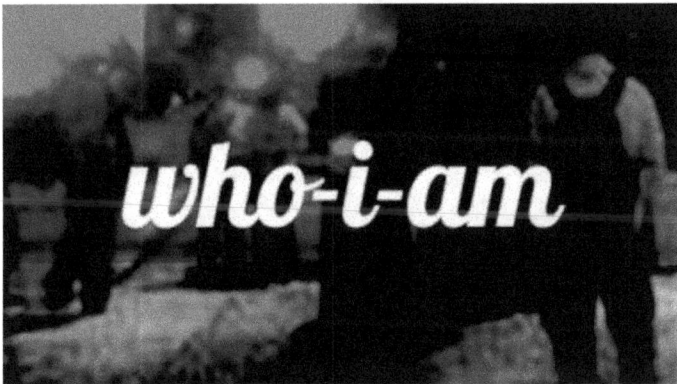

About the Author

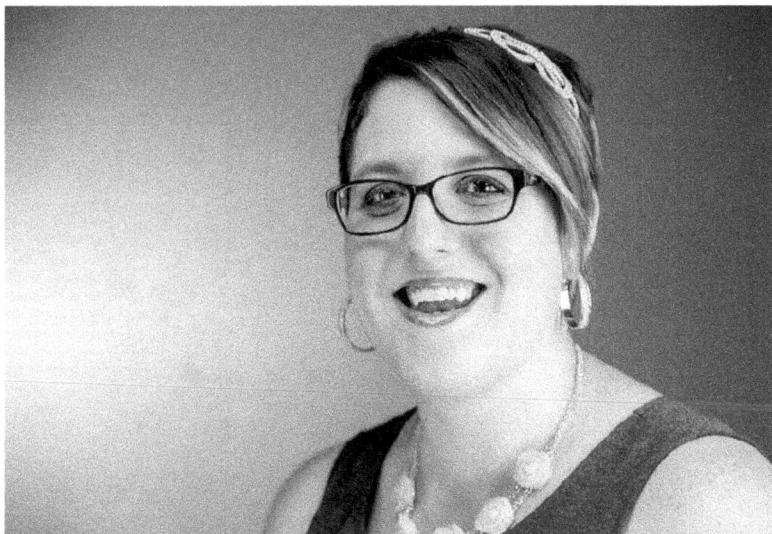

Shannon Ketchum has been a wife since 2003, fur mom, sister, introvert and most importantly in love with Jesus! She has been dealing with infertility since 2003 due to endometriosis, hypothyroidism, PCOS and a pelvic spasm condition. She's believing God for her promised miracle children! Shannon is the founder of *Embrace Bravery*, a support ministry for women with infertility, a blogger, author and speaker. In *Embrace Bravery*, women bravely embrace the difficult journey of infertility in a safe place by learning how to trust God while growing deeper in relationship with Him. She is passionate for women to break free from the brokenness of infertility and experience Jesus in a whole new way.

Shannon would love to share her heart with your ministry or at your event. Book Shannon Ketchum to speak at your event or conference. All requests for speaking engagements should be submitted at **embracebravery. com/speaking.**

Contact Shannon:
embracebravery.com
shannon@embracebravery.com
FB Page: facebook.com/embracebraverynow
FB Group: facebook.com/groups/embracebravery
IG & TW: @embracebravery

www.ingramcontent.com/pod-product-compliance
Lightning Source LLC
Chambersburg PA
CBHW071340290326
41933CB00040B/1827